DECOMPRESS

Live Your Life Free From Back Pain

How Non-Surgical Spinal Decompression
Can Eliminate Your Back Pain And
Save You From Spine Surgery Or
Reliance On Medications

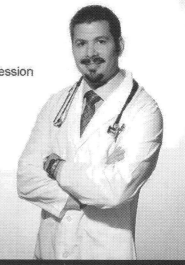

Dr. Leonard Molczan

Order this book online at www.trafford.com
or email orders@trafford.com

Most Trafford titles are also available at major online book retailers.

Printed in the United States of America.

ISBN: 978-1-4669-1467-4 (sc)
ISBN: 978-1-4669-1469-8 (hc)
ISBN: 978-1-4669-1468-1 (e)

Library of Congress Control Number: 2012902726

Trafford rev. 02/23/2012

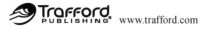 www.trafford.com

North America & international
toll-free: 1 888 232 4444 (USA & Canada)
phone: 250 383 6864 ♦ fax: 812 355 4082

Acknowledgements

There are many to thank for their personal contributions towards this work. Please allow me a moment to single out a few here:

I would like to thank Lance Liberti of Prime Business Management for his guidance and assistance. Lance's tremendous knowledge of VAX-D and the spinal decompression industry, along with his business acumen and his expertise in marketing have been invaluable for this project.

I also wish to thank Dr. Alan Dyer and Dr. Larry Dyer for bringing the technology of VAX-D to us. I know it wasn't easy, but there is no way of telling how many lives you have touched through your work.

Thanks are due to Dr. John Boren and Dr. Patrick Gentempo. Dr. John Boren's mentorship fully opened my eyes to surviving the business struggles associated with managing a non-surgical spinal decompression specialty clinic. Dr. Patrick Gentempo's mentorship has made me a better doctor, a better businessman and a better human being. Thanks are further due to Dr. James Chestnut. His understanding of the human ecosystem has made us all healthier.

Thanks to Dr. Bryan Hawley for his help during the early years of my practice. His mentorship was irreplaceable. Thanks should additionally be given to Dr. Frank Liberti, although we did not get the chance to work together, I'd like to acknowledge your vast efforts in advancing the field of non-surgical spinal decompression. Thanks to Dr. Jason Lazeroff for our weekly lunch meetings. They have meant the world to me. I could not have gotten through the stressful times without your friendship.

Special thanks to Dr. D.D. Palmer and Dr. B.J. Palmer, for their amazing contribution to the world.

Finally, words alone cannot express the debt of gratitude I owe to Leonard and Norma Molczan, my parents, for their support and love. You are the best anyone could ask for.

Foreword

The total cost of low back pain exceeds one hundred billion dollars per year in the United States alone. More than half of these costs are related to lost wages and decreased productivity at work. It has been reported that surgical treatment for low back pain has grown more widespread over the past twenty years, and may be overused. The analysis of long-term data suggests that invasive high cost surgeries do not afford better outcomes when compared to conservative treatments with their approach to low back pain. The research demonstrates similar outcomes for non-operative approaches over several domains, including patient symptoms, quality of life, and the use of healthcare resources.

The results reported in the literature therefore mandate an effort to continue to develop the best non-surgical approach to the long-term management of chronic back pain. The old adage seems to be true: If you have your health, you have everything; If you don't have your health and you live with chronic pain, the quality of your life is drastically affected and almost all daily activities and pleasures will often take a back seat.

I found this out more than 25 years ago after developing several herniated discs in my back. My parents, Dr. Allan Dyer and mother Dr. Natalie Dyer were also afflicted with chronic herniated discs and being in the medical business, none of us wanted surgery; so necessity became the mother of invention. They had developed a crude frame and boat-winch type device to use around the house that would apply tension and stretch the spine. You had to wear garbage bags over your pants so that the lower body would slide over the carpet while the upper body remained stationary while you held on to a crossbar. However crude, the device worked like a miracle. Soon we had all our friends in the neighborhood coming over for treatments. VAX-D (vertebral axial decompression) Therapy has literally kept all of us from going to surgery for more than twenty years now.

As we developed this into a pneumatic device, early clinical studies demonstrated that it was indeed possible to lower the pressure within the disc with this device. Dr. Gustavo Ramos, a neurosurgeon associated with the University of Texas, performed intradiscal pressure studies that helped define the treatment parameters and shaped the protocols for VAX-D Therapy.

Many people who suffer from chronic back and neck pain have already seen multiple disciplines such as physical therapy, prescriptions, injections, and even surgery to no avail. In our common daily activities we subject our bodies to all sorts of postures that increase the pressure with the spinal disc. Postures like sitting at a desk looking at a computer screen. This might seem innocuous, yet sitting in a flexed positon certainly increases the disc pressure and stress on the spine. This book looks at these everyday activities to show just what is happening in the disc.

This book is a presentation to inform people about VAX-D Therapy, still one of the most under utilized treatments in the field of back pain. The thrust at VAX-D Medical Technologies has been in the clinical arena and not one of marketing. Not only is the public not that aware of the treatment, but many general physicians and specialists are not aware of the benefits. In *DECOMPRESS: Live Your Life Free From Back Pain*, Dr. Molczan answers the question that many patients ask: "So why haven't I heard of VAX-D before?"

Many times in medicine change comes slowly; and the system is now driven by the healthcare and insurance industries, so the monetary concerns are often a deciding factor in what treatments become mainstream medicine. A physician once told me it can take 30-40 years after inception, before a treatment is universally accepted into mainstream medicine.

While surgery is a viable option for many patients, the fact remains that the bulk of low back pain patients are just not surgical candidates.

Dr. Molczan has been treating low back pain for twelve years, and has focused solely on VAX-D Therapy for three. This book was written to help disseminate the information that desparately needs to get out. Dr. Molczan writes a 'call to action' and challenges his readers and his patients to take responsibity for their own life, look at the clinical studies (for this or other potential treatments) and then, take action.

The patient must do their homework because there are a lot of back pain treatments out there that are heavily marketed with "hype" with little or no clinical studies; or that are twenty year old traction systems that are re-packaged and re-marketed as spinal decompression. Today, people do their research with internet searches. Look for this original treatment system and base your decision on clinical research. VAX-D Therapy studies can be found at www.vaxd.com.

The causes of back pain are often multi-factorial and not just a result of one single pathology. We are all fighting old age which brings arthritis, dehydration of tissues and stenosis from chronic inflammation; coupled with the fact that there is a restricted blood supply to the discs themselves and also trauma from years of abuse and yet we try to recapture our youth.

We're not sure why VAX-D Therapy works as well as it does. It's the only non-surgical treatment known to lower the pressure inside the disc. If we look at the laws of physics, creating a negative intradiscal pressure creates a diffusion gradient across the vertebral bone end plate where the disc gets its blood supply. This would allow for the exchange of more fluids than the rest of the twenty four hours a day when the disc is compressed. This exchange of fluid brings in the building blocks of living tissue: oxygen, fluids, and nutrients. It would also allow for the reduction of unwanted catabolites that build up within the disc, such as lactic acid, that would not normally be reduced with the disc under compression.

We believe all of this simply reduces the inflammation within the disc and the surrounding structures, which helps the body to heal.

VAX-D Therapy has in itself evolved over the past twenty years and has been refined with today's technology of computer science. Due to advances in motion control and new software programs, today's VAX-D Therapy equipment is easier to use and much more accurate that it was at its inception.

VAX-D Therapy has addressed an old medical hypothesis that if we could successfully lower the pressure within the discs of the spine, then conditions would be created where the discs and spine as a whole could heal. For many patients, the effects of VAX-D Therapy are both immediate and long lasting. If the patient should reinjure their disc, they can simply take another course of treatment.

The mission of VAX-D Medical Technologies and Dr. Molczan's personal lifework is to make VAX-D Therapy available to all patients, in all communities, the standard of care for the treatment of chronic low back pain. VAX-D Therapy is a safe, cost effective, non-surgical treatment that offers new hope for the millions of people who suffer from low back pain everyday. I guess VAX-D Therapy could be viewed as, "Chicken Soup For Your Back."

- Lawrence Dyer, M.D. {VAX-D Medical Technologies}

Table of Contents

Introduction

On any given day, back pain affects 31 million adults and accounts for 3.6 million outpatient visits in the United States. This is second only to pregnancy. It has been reported that more money is spent on back pain than any other condition. To be more specific, pain associated to the low back is estimated at over 100 billion dollars in expenditures annually. This represents one quarter of the annual health care budget. Back pain is pandemic. Navigating through what is fact or merely opinions regarding back pain and how best to address it can be a daunting task for anyone.

There are many causes for Low Back Pain (LBP) and as a result, volumes have been written on the subject. Some books serve as clinical texts to understand the many conditions that trigger the pain response. Other books act as a guide through the multitude of treatment options. This book is presented as an alternative treatment for the most common causes of chronic LBP. This alternative is non-surgical and in most cases, does not require the use of medication. This alternative continues to be proven effective in study after study and has a track record of success in cases that have been unresponsive to other treatments. However, this alternative treatment is not typically offered as an option by your primary care physician and thus, it is unfortunately underutilized. The technology used has helped thousands of patients find the relief they had been hoping for. This alternative treatment is called Non-Surgical Spinal Decompression or more specifically, VAX-D (Vertebral Axial Decompression) Therapy.

VAX-D Therapy has been touted as a medical breakthrough, the fountain of youth for your spine, and by some a miracle. The technology of VAX-D literally reverses the effect gravity has on the spine, allowing the human body to do what it always strive to do: maintain homeostasis (balance) and heal itself.

If you are reading this book, you are probably experiencing chronic LBP or know someone who suffers from chronic LBP and want to help them. As a doctor, I am naturally sympathetic to patients who are experiencing pain and want to respond swiftly to treat their condition with the highest degree of efficacy. As a former VAX-D Therapy patient myself, I can empathize with patients who suffer chronic LBP. I want to share my personal success story and the testimonials of other satisfied VAX-D Therapy patients all over the world and offer you hope that you too, can Live Your Life Free From Back Pain. Hopefully, before you're finished reading this book, you will be able to decide if the solution for your low back pain (or neck pain) can be found through VAX-D.

Who Should Read This Book?

Chronic Low Back Pain is defined as pain lasting more than three months. Most soft tissues heal within six to twelve weeks marking the threshold. The treatments for acute LBP lasting up to three months are as numerous as are the causes. This book has not been written with the acute patient in mind. It will however, benefit the chronic LBP patient or the chronic LBP patient with an acute relapse whom often report: "I've tried everything and nothing worked."

My office, Pennsylvania Spinal Care, specializes in the treatment of chronic LBP as well as chronic neck pain. The majority of my patients often believe their LBP is beyond help. Patients' stories reported in my consultation room are frequently similar: "Years ago, I had my first experience with back pain while just bending over. I heard a pop and I could not stand up straight. My doctor gave me muscle relaxers, but they didn't work. I tried massage, acupuncture, chiropractic . . . Those made it feel better for a little while but it didn't last. My doctor sent me to a pain management specialist who gave me three injections. I got a few weeks of pain relief but the pain came back even worse than before. I had surgery next. It didn't work. I am still in pain every day. I don't think there is anything you can do for me."

I would love nothing more than to be able to help every individual that seeks my consultation. Unfortunately, this just isn't possible. There are many individuals I have to refer to other specialists. Between 10%-15% of my consult patients are not candidates for VAX-D Therapy.

In order for a patient to qualify for my treatment, I utilize a questionnaire, take a complete medical history, review prior diagnostic testing results and perform a brief exam. There are many factors that go into the clinical decision-making process but I rely heavily on the diagnostic testing component, mainly Magnetic Resonance Imaging (MRI) and Computerized Tomography (CT). MRI and CT exams are two diagnostic studies that show an actual soft tissue picture from inside the body. Both exams come with a pathology report written by a Radiologist. If you have had one of these tests, take a moment to review your report and look for the diagnoses outlined in Table 1. These conditions could indicate that you may be a candidate for VAX-D Therapy:

Table 1

Bulging/ Herniated Disc	Disc Protrusion	Extruded Disc	Disc Degeneration
Degenerative Disc Disease	Loss of Disc Signal	Disc Desiccation	IDD
Facet Arthrosis	Spondylolisthesis	Foraminal Stenosis	Sciatica
Spinal Stenosis (secondary to disc herniation)		Nerve Root Compression	

Remarkable success rates have been reported in treating all of the above conditions with VAX-D Therapy. If you have any of these conditions appearing on your report, I encourage you to continue reading. I can assure you that these conditions can be treated successfully and you do not have to "learn to live with it."

I'm not just the doctor, I'm also a patient!

At age 38, I began to experience a disconcerting symptom. My left testicle started to go numb. It felt as though it had something wrapped completely around it and lightly squeezing on it. It wasn't excruciating, just constant pressure.

As you can guess, I initially assumed the worst. Approaching 40, insidious onset of testicular pain . . . Oh my God, I have testicular cancer!

Fortunately, I was working at a wellness center and one of the chiropractors there said, "Len, let me check your low back for subluxation." As he laid my torso over his fist high on my lower back and impulsed his body weight onto mine, I felt the most exhilarating, electric shock for a fraction of a second. Then, it was like the light switch was turned off and my testicular pain was completely gone.

I've received hundreds, if not thousands, of adjustments by that time but never one quite like this. It was an Ah-ha moment for me. The pain was definitely due to pressure on a spinal nerve being referred into my groin. MRI confirmed diffuse spinal degeneration throughout my lumbar region.

Unfortunately however, as amazing as that original adjustment was, the pain in my groin would continually return within a day or two after each adjustment. That's when I learned more about VAX-D Therapy and found that I didn't have to suffer anymore. I received my treatment and subsequent certification as a practitioner then, opened my first VAX-D clinic near my hometown of Philadelphia, PA.

I became a believer because I experienced it firsthand. I am still pain free after 4 plus years!

Dr. Leonard Molczan

There Is No Such Thing As A Cure All

VAX-D Therapy is not a panacea for all causes of chronic LBP. I wish this were true. I wish that I could help every chronic LBP patient, with every condition, every time. But, it would be disingenuous of me to suggest that. However, for those who have conditions considered responsive through the use of Non-Surgical Spinal Decompression, there is hardly a better option to ensure a successful pain free outcome than VAX-D Therapy.

I encourage you to review the evidence-based research of the most frequently utilized treatments from the non-specific category of musculoskeletal back pain causes. Their findings may surprise you. References for these studies are provided for you to have easy access in the event you would like to perform research of your own.

> "I went from a daily runner to not being able to walk. After completing treatment, I was able to run 9 miles and I no longer have to take any meds."
>
> Tracy H.

Chapter 1

> "I had back surgery about 18 years ago by one of the best doctors, but about a year ago I started experiencing severe pain. My pain was a 10 on a scale of 1-10. By my fourth session, it went down to about an 8 and from the 12th on, I felt amazing."
>
> Gail H.

Sobering Statistics

The Basics

Chronic LBP affects 31 million adults at any given time.

One in every five people has chronic or severe back pain that is affecting their quality of life.

Experts estimate that as many as 80% of the population will experience a back problem at some time in their lives.

One third of all American adults have experienced back pain in the last 30 days. Back pain is the leading reason for visits to physicians.

Back pain is the leading reason for visits to Neurologists.

Back pain is the leading reason for visits to Orthopedists.

Back pain is the second reason for hospitalization, pregnancy being number one.

Overexertion accounts for 60% of all low back problems.

Most cases of back pain are mechanical or non-organic; they are not caused by serious conditions such as inflammatory arthritis, infection, fracture or cancer.

Back pain should not be considered a normal part of aging. It is a chronic condition that calls for lifestyle changes just as lifestyle changes are essential in patients suffering from arthritis and diabetes.

Ten million Americans initially develop low back pain as a result of overexertion or strain injury.

According to the National Center for Health Statistics, reported rates of LBP are higher in Caucasians than in any other ethnic group.

The incidence of LBP is higher in females than in males and more common in adults older than 25 years of age.

The prevalence of chronic low back pain in the U.S. is 27% with an onset likely occurring between the ages of 45 and 64.

Each year, approximately 3.6 million outpatient visits in the United States are attributed to chronic LBP.

Many experts believe the problem has been "over-medicalized."

Work Facts

Back Pain is the #1 worker's compensation injury.

One in 20 workers will suffer a low back injury every year.

Back pain is one of the most common reasons for work days missed. Back pain is the second most common reason for visits to the doctor's office, outnumbered only by upper-respiratory infections.

More sick days are lost to back pain than any other condition, over 550 million days annually.

One-half of all working Americans admit to having back pain symptoms each year.

LBP is also regarded as the most common cause of job-related disability, resulting in significant societal burden. Indirect costs related to LBP total $30 billion annually, with approximately 2% of the U.S. workforce compensated for back injuries.

Americans spend at least $50 billion each year on back pain. This total represents only the more readily identifiable costs for medical care, worker's compensation payments and time lost from work. It does not include costs associated with lost personal income due to acquired physical limitation resulting from a back problem and lost employer productivity due to employee medical absence.

According to the American Chronic Pain Association, 11.7 million people reported that they are "impaired" by back pain and 2.6 million reported they are permanently disabled by back pain.

Chronic low back pain accounted for 23% ($8.8 billion) of total worker's compensation payments in 1995.

The Money

More money is spent on chronic LBP than any other condition.

One quarter of the annual health care budget is spent on pain, primarily back pain, over $100 billion annually.

Each year, Americans spend an estimated $24 billion on treatments for back pain. This total does not include missed time from work.

Back Pain Expenditures:	in Dollars
Office Visits	11.1 billion
Hospitalization	4.5 billion
Prescription Drugs	3.9 billion
Outpatient Visits	4.7 billion
Emergency Room	1.1 billion

Lower Back Surgery

51% of all back surgery is unnecessary.

53% of all lumbar back surgeries fail to produce relief of symptoms.

Morbidity and mortality rates, as well as hospital charges, increase with age among persons having lumbar spine surgery.

"The rising costs and the growth in the number of back surgeries is a good example of why health care expenditures are more than double inflation."

"There's a raging debate going on right now. The issue of whether spinal fusion or back surgery in general is overused was part of the discussions at the North American Spine Society meeting in Philadelphia where officials say that the questions about back surgery have been raised by doctors themselves."

"Some doctors may argue as to whether more and costlier procedures benefit patients. And, when asked if patients are better off, nobody knows."

There is a major shift to spinal fusion procedures that use expensive mechanical devices to fuse diseased vertebrae together. "It's expensive and has not resulted in significantly better outcomes."

There is no evidence that spinal fusion, one of the most common operations for low back problems, is superior to other surgical procedures for common degenerative conditions of the spine.

Patients who undergo spinal fusions have more complications, longer hospital stays and higher hospital charges than do patients undergoing other types of back surgery.

Chapter 2

"You must take personal responsibility. You cannot change the circumstances, the seasons, or the wind, but you can change yourself."

-Jim Rohn {American business philosopher}

A Call To Action

Many of the people who visit my office have lived with chronic LBP for years. Oftentimes, they show up for their initial consultation with personal experiences that cause them to challenge educational information presented to them. There are those that are doubtful anyone can help them in their particular case. I don't blame them. Some have been through many failed treatment attempts. Others are just frightened when their bodies respond in a manner alien to what they remember to be "normal." Regardless, their willingness to show up for a consultation proves that they believe there is a solution out there. I like to remind them that a solution exists for every problem. No matter how badly things seem to be given your individual circumstances I beg you, please press on. You will find the answers you are looking for. You've heard the old proverb, "When the student is ready, the teacher will appear." More apropos to our discussion is the saying: "When the patient is ready, the treatment will appear." Hang in there and stay the course. You will find a solution for your chronic LBP whether it lies within these pages or beyond.

Take Responsibility

In his book *Success Principles*, Jack Canfield, also known for his *Chicken Soup for the Soul* books, lists 64 ideas to help you achieve success in any endeavor you may undertake. Principle #1: "Take 100% Responsibility for your Life." I for one think it is very telling that he chooses this concept to be not somewhat important, but the most important on his entire list. You must take control of your life, your happiness and your health. The brightest minds agree that when you are faced with a challenge or crisis, it is you that must take responsibility for it. Unfortunately, you are often the one that must find a solution for yourself. The same is true regarding your health. Of course, you can and should seek out doctors for their advice. They are highly trained professionals and there is no replacement for their experience. However, sometimes patients just don't find the answers they are looking for despite the best efforts of their doctors.

James L. Chestnut B.Ed, MSc., D.C., considered the foremost expert on the science of human wellness, proved through evidence-based research from the most respected journals in the world that it is not bad bugs, bad luck or bad genes that cause the chronic health issues plaguing our society today, but rather our own bad choices. Our lifestyle choices have clearly impacted our health. We continually see evidence of this all around us more and more every day. If you're left with problems unresolved after following your doctor's advice, find another doctor or seek alternatives to mainstream care. Whatever you decide, it is important to stay determined not to give up looking for the answer best suited for you. Keep searching for the solution until you find success. If your pain affects the quality of your life you owe it to yourself to continue the quest.

I can often be heard in my consultation room telling prospective patients that I will only work with them if they are 100% committed to resolving their back pain. If someone tells me that they are 99% or less, I ask them to return when they reach 100%. This is not for effect. I recognize that they are the ones that will have to "do the work" so to speak. They must be actively engaged in their rehabilitation. They have to commit to showing up for their appointments, follow their care plan explicitly and carry out the many additional recommendations that will benefit their health. I refer to individuals who actively engage in achieving and maintaining their own health as Pro-Active Regarding Health or P.R.H. P.R.H.'s are usually physically fit, they eat healthy most of the time, they do not smoke, they consume little to no alcohol and they smile frequently. They find solutions for themselves in most areas of their lives. They feel great, regularly. They understand the concept of wellness and they live it.

Individuals who are less engaged in achieving and maintaining their own health are Re-Active Regarding Health or R.R.H. R.R.H's are typically overweight, eat whatever they want, smoke, drink alcohol and are always putting out fires. They respond to health emergencies only. They believe in better living through chemistry and live out of their medicine cabinets. They rarely feel good. They do not understand the concept of wellness and seldom express it.

Healing Is A Process

The western culture is one that lives for instant gratification and quick fixes. Yet, throughout our history that fact has been shown to be detrimental to many of the things that we do, especially when it comes to the health of our people. Healing is a process. By definition, there is no process on the planet that does not require time. I can show you through the research that the quick fixes as they relate specifically to chronic LBP are simply not the best options for long term benefit.

Taking an anti-inflammatory often helps with acute injury relief such as a muscle strain following rigorous snow shoveling. But, chronic LBP lasts longer than 90-days. If the pain persists past three months, clearly, the use of anti-inflammatory needs to be reevaluated.

Degeneration also is a process. It is logical then that the process of healing degenerative conditions also takes time. Much like investing in long-term conservative stocks or bonds, slow and steady usually wins the race and consistently produces calculable returns for the investor. Investing in "get rich quick" schemes rarely work out the way you wish them to. Invest for long-term health and achieve the wellness you deserve to experience.

Play The Odds

I am not a gambling man. I always acknowledge the simple fact that the odds favor the house. Yet, there exist professional gamblers who know how to swing the odds slightly in their favor with enough proficiency to turn this skill into a career. I like to remember that when I think of health.

There are no guarantees in life. Likewise, there are no guarantees regarding your health. You can be a marathon runner and still die reasonably young from a heart attack like Jim Fixx, and others. In contrast, one can smoke cigarettes their entire life and never manifest lung cancer. However, despite the controversial cover-up from the leading tobacco companies, we now accept the fact, along with the surgeon general's warning on every box, that cigarettes do indeed cause lung cancer. Smoking prevalence has decreased as a result.

Participating in healthy activities won't guarantee that you stay healthy. However, the odds increase with every healthy habit you routinely perform.

I always try to stack the chips in my favor. Healthy choices will undoubtedly increase the odds for a healthy outcome. If there are steps that you can take to increase the odds of a favorable result, should you not make the effort? I certainly can't presume to answer that question for anyone other than for myself. The responsibility is always on the individual. I like to remind my patients that they can oftentimes be the crucial difference in their own success. VAX-D Therapy, as you will come to find, is a healthy habit that puts the body under optimal conditions to do what it always strive to do: heal itself.

P.R.H.'s (Pro-Active Regarding Health) aren't always immune from chronic LBP and many still end up at my office in pain. It's more frequently from trauma or overexertion than it is from degenerative pathology. However, in my experience, I can assure you that it's the R.R.H.'s (Re-Active Regarding Health) that are by far more susceptible to suffer chronic LBP. Furthermore, R.R.H.'s typically respond more slowly to treatment than do their counterparts.

There are many things that individuals can do to help themselves when they take control of their actions and lifestyle choices.

Probability Is Not Absolute

Probability denotes only the relative frequency of occurrence of a particular outcome. It is not an absolute!

When your doctor gives a prognosis, the outcome is not definitive. It is a statistic derived from looking at cases of patients with similar conditions and the outcome that most experienced. There is no definite way for that doctor to know which side of the statistic a patient will be on and there are numerous examples of patients beating the odds. Even in the worst-case scenarios, people have triumphed.

Certain types of cancers, such as pancreatic cancer, have around 90% mortality rate. Nevertheless, many patients outlive their prognosis. Rabies has a 99% mortality rate. If left untreated, most victims will die. There have been millions of deaths recorded from untreated rabies since record keeping began. However, as deadly as it is, there have been four documented cases of recovery.

Never Lose Hope

Hope exists for those who suffer chronic LBP. A strong belief in any treatment's effectiveness increases the chances of it being effective. Hence, the "Placebo Effect." What you may not know is that the exact opposite is also true. A strong belief in something "not working for me" will surely decrease the chances of it working. This is known as the "Nocebo Effect." There is an entire branch of science, Psychoneuroimmunology (PNI), that deals with the way in which the Body-Mind functions. The research in this field is irrefutable. If you choose to remain hopeful and belief you can be healed, you too can Live Your Life Free From Back Pain!

"Once you choose hope, anything's possible."

-Christopher Reeve {Superman}

Chapter 3

Etiology: The Science Of Causation

There are many causes for chronic LBP ranging from psychological to malignancy, and everything else in between. It would be a bit too onerous to read through them all. Therefore, I would like to keep our focus on the conditions that have been shown to respond to VAX-D Therapy and limit our discussion of those outside the scope of care for this treatment.

Specific Causes are, as a whole, considered outside the scope of VAX-D Therapy. These include congenital, infectious, malignant, metabolic and traumatic. Examples of Specific Causes are:

- Congenital Spinal Stenosis
- Osteoporosis
- Ankylosing Spondylitis
- Fracture

Also important to note is that **Red Flag Symptoms** can be concomitant with back pain. I would direct you to your family doctor or your local emergency room in the event of these symptoms, as they could indicate very serious conditions needing immediate attention. Examples of Red Flag Symptoms are:

- Back pain associated with illness, fever, or rapid weight loss.
- Back pain associated with bowel and/or bladder incontinence.
- Back pain following a significant trauma with risk of fracture.

- Back pain in patients with a history of cancer or family history of cancer.

Pain can also be felt in the lower back while the area of pathology actually exists elsewhere in the body. This is known as referred pain. The referral pain patterns below are contraindicated for VAX-D Therapy.

Referral Pain

Abdominal Aortic Aneurysm (AAA)	A dilation, or ballooning out, of the abdominal aorta supplying blood to the abdomen and lower extremities.
Gastrointestinal Disorders	Disorders pertaining to the gut and digestion.
Hip Pathology	Disease of the hip joint itself.
Gynecological Disorders	Female reproductive disorders.
Genitourinary Disorders	Disorders of genitalia or urinary system.

The **Non-Specific Causes** are far more prevalent and include the musculoskeletal conditions below:

Mechanical

Strain	Microtrauma, over-stretching, or tearing of muscles. Typically due to overexertion.
Sprain	Microtrauma, overstretching, or tearing of the ligaments that hold bone to bone. Typically due to rapid, unexpected movements.
Subluxations	Spinal misalignments causing nervous interference.
Trigger Points	Highly sensitive knots within muscles. They typically radiate pain to other areas of the body.

Bulging Discs	Slight compression of spinal discs causing a bulging of the exterior.
Herniated Discs Slipped Discs Ruptured Discs Pinched Nerve	Moderate compression of spinal discs where the internal pressure causes the interior matrix to break through the outer bands of the disc. The nucleus of the disc spills out through the broken fibers.
Degenerative Disc Disease	Aging process when spinal discs diminish in size and lose vital water and other nutrients.
Facet Syndrome	Osteoarthritic changes to connecting joints of the spine causing pain.
Spinal Stenosis	Narrowing of the spaces within the spinal column. Typically associated with radiating pain down an extremity.
Spondylolisthesis	Forward slippage of one vertebra over top of another.
Posture	Poor posture, slouching, or otherwise placing your body into positions that produce greater load forces than biomechanically designed for.
Obesity	Being overweight which produces excess load for your body to carry.
Pregnancy	Carrying extra weight from a developing fetus that puts an excessive load onto an expecting mother.
Lack of Fitness	Loss of muscle tone causing weakness and less ability for the body to support itself.
Tension Myositis Syndrome	Psychologically induced back pain.
Ischemia	Lack of oxygen caused by a restriction of blood supply to any tissue, in this case the muscles of the lower back.

Of these causes of chronic LBP, the following are Non-Treatable Conditions (contraindications for VAX-D):

- Spinal Tumors
- Vertebral Fractures
- Osteoporosis
- Severe Medical Conditions
- Pregnancy
- Ankylosing Spondylitis
- Spinal Fusion with retained hardware
- Spinal Infections
- Spinal Stenosis (hard tissue growth/hypertrophy)

Etiology: The Statistics

The epidemiological study below was conducted in 1996 to establish the diagnoses contributing to the chronic LBP epidemic. The overwhelming majority of causes reported were, as outlined in the previous chapter, mechanical in nature. Most of the cases below can be treated successfully with VAX-D Therapy.

Final Diagnosis in 2,374 Chronic Low Back Pain Patients Participating in the National Low Back Pain Study

Diagnosis	Percentage of Cases
Herniated Disc	36.7
Myofascial Pain	19.6
Spinal Stenosis	14.0
Lumbar Spondylosis	12.2
Osteoarthritis Root Compression	8.7
Unknown Etiology	8.5
Spondylolisthesis	7.3
Discogenic Pain	6.1
Facet Arthropathy	4.8
Lumbar Instability	3.6
Spondylosis	3.1

Scoliosis	3.1
Pain with Psychiatric Component	2.2
Compression Fracture	1.9
Epidural Fibrosis	1.3
Epineural Fibrosis	0.8
Arachnoiditis	0.6
Spina Bifida	0.5
Other Diagnosis	5.1

(Adapted from Long DM, Ben Debba M. Torgerson WS. et al. *Persistent back pain and sciatica in the United States: Patient charastic.* J Spinai Discord 1996.9:40-58).

It's rare, in my office at least, that I review an MRI and it reveals only one abnormal finding or diagnosis, affecting only one level of the spine. It happens occasionally in the young adult population following an acute trauma such as sports injury or motor vehicle accident. But more often than not, I find diffuse spinal degeneration affecting the middle aged and the elderly. Their MRI shows multiple abnormal findings throughout multiple levels of the spine.

There are three forms of stress: physical, chemical and emotional. The majority of stressors on the spine that contribute to its decay are physical in nature. Addressing the physical mechanism is then paramount. It is only logical to address those physical problems with a physical remedy. Yes, there are components of chemical stressors on and around the spinal unit and yes, emotional components as well. However, treating a predominantly physical problem using only chemical interventions (NSAID's, Corticosteroids, etc.) or emotional counseling (treatment for Tension Myositis Syndrome) while completely neglecting the physical component is a mistake and one made far too often.

Better still, is a treatment approach that addresses all three forms of stress on your spine to increase the odds of a successful outcome. The use of pharmacological agents such as oral steroids, NSAID, muscle relaxants, analgesics and even calcium supplements is sometimes included in a well managed VAX-D Therapy care plan to induce a relaxed state during the treatment process. My treatment rooms mimic a spa experience and create an environment for optimal relaxation and healing.

Similar to many spinal decompression centers, my clinic advertises the "Non-Surgical/Non-Drug" aspect of the therapy. However, my clinic has a team of doctors ready to potentially address all three forms of stress affecting a given patient and the multiple components to managing a care plan. I have seen thousands of spines over the years and no two are the same. I try to address individual needs and individual responses to care throughout the healing process.

Again following the rule of probability, PRH's may want to try to avoid some of the known risk factors for chronic LBP whenever possible. If you can't avoid them all together, try to limit exposure or be mindful that injury could occur and pay close attention to ergonomics, etc.

Risk Factors For Mechanical (non-specific) Causes Of Chronic LBP:

- Heavy physical labor
- Frequent twisting and bending
- Lifting and forceful movements
- Repetitive movements
- Vibration
- Smoking
- Improper body mechanics
- Insufficient exercise
- Prolonged sitting or driving
- Obesity
- Spinal abnormalities
- Genetic predisposition
- Pregnancy
- Psychosocial stress
- Psychological stress

- Health paradigm
- Aging

"Every morning I woke up in excruciating pain. If I got down on the floor I would not be able to get back up. After 10 sessions of VAX-D treatment, zero pain. I stood tall like I have not done in a long time."

Bob E.

Chapter 4

"It's a good thing we have gravity, or else when birds died they'd just stay right up there. Hunters would be all confused."

-Steven Wright {comedian}

Gravity's Effects On Our Spine

Gravity! You only need look upon the faces of the elderly to see how the unrelenting pull towards the earth weakens and distorts our body's tissues over time. Compression of the spinal joints is where some of the most significant effects can be measured. Over your lifetime you can lose up to two inches in height due to the force of gravity. A closer look at the individual segment of the spine reveals how such dramatic degeneration progresses.

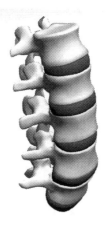

Normal Spinal Column
Healthy Intervertebral Discs In Gray

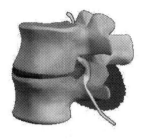
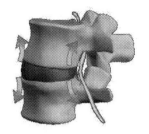

Degenerated Spinal Column   **Opening Up The Joints Is Needed**

The spine is composed of 33 vertebrae (individual spinal bones). Starting from the bottom-up, there are four coccogeal bones that are usually fused in two followed by five sacral bones that are fused together to form part of the pelvis. There are five lumbar vertebrae that make up the low-back, 12-thoracic vertebrae in the mid-back, and seven cervical vertebrae in the neck. The movements of the cervical, thoracic and lumbar vertebrae are independent of each other and move freely on their own. Sandwiched between these bones, with exception of the first and second cervical, are the soft shock absorbing, load bearing intervertebral discs.

Similar to a jelly donut, the spinal disc has a flat, round exterior case containing jelly in the middle. The outer portion, or annulus, is made up of concentric rings of collagen fibers. Think of rolling a magazine into a tube, the pages representing the fibers. The inner nucleus (the jelly) has the consistency of toothpaste and bears the load of the axial weight.

Water: The Essential Nutrient

"If there is magic on this planet, it is contained in water."

-Loran Eisely {Novelist}

35

Water content is vital to a healthy spinal disc. The outer bands of the annulus are approximately 60-65% water. The inner Nucleus is 80-85% water. The disc nucleus is responsible for supporting the axial load. Dehydration of the disc causes a shifting of that load onto the annulus. This creates stress, as the annulus is not designed to bear excessive loading. The disc subsequently bulges under the pressure. The dehydration of the annulus causes the outer bands to become weaker, thus tearing and eventually leading to a full-blown Disc Herniation.

"You can't blame gravity for falling in love."

-Albert Einstein {Nobel Prize Physicist}

Gravity's constant squeeze on our bodies causes them to dehydrate during the course of the day. Depending on the axial load time (such as sitting upright or standing still), the loss of water can add up to an overall loss of ½ inch to ¾ inch height per day. Fortunately, the discs rehydrate overnight when the pressure decreases. However, as you age, less and less rehydration occurs. Degeneration usually begins with decreased blood supply after your teen years. The average height loss is ½ inch for every 20 years after skeletal maturity.

The disc relies almost solely on hydrostatic motion for proper nutrient or fluid exchange to take place. Trauma such as increased postural stress and a sedentary lifestyle accelerates degeneration. The internal environment of the disc also degrades when this dehydration continues. This process is called Internal Disc Disruption (IDD). When IDD progresses to the outer third of the annular fibers, the individual will most likely experience tearing and thus pain. There is also the possibility of the chemical degradation process causing radicular pain (sciatica) without actual mechanical pressure on the nerve root next to the disc.

You might be thinking to yourself that people are naturally going to degenerate and shrink. While it's true that our bodies do "wear out" over the course of our lifetime, the fact is that our bodies are designed for work, and a lot of it. We are hunter-gatherers. We are made to be able to walk, lift, bend, and stretch all day. Our Stone Age hunter-gatherer ancestors were as physically fit as today's most elite athletes. The degree of degeneration that is pandemic in western society today is huge when compared to the degeneration found in the fossil records of hunter-gatherers. Our primarily sedentary lifestyle, lack of physical fitness and poor diet prevents us from experiencing optimal health. The human body is not built to sit in front of computers eight hours a day in poor, unsupportive postures, eating fast-foods only to head home to sit in front of the new flat screen TV. Spines are made of joints. Joints are designed for movement. The less movement they get, the worse they function. Period.

Later we will discuss in detail the recommendations R.R.H.'s can take to become P.R.H.'s. You can stack the odds in your favor and lessen the probability of a degenerative condition advancing to the point at which it will negatively affect your quality of life.

> "My quality of life was horrible. The day-to-day pain was almost unbearable. Upon completion of treatment, I was able to play 18 holes of golf, pain free."
>
> Brent F.

Chapter 5

So What Is VAX-D?

VAX-D Theory

Vertebral Axial Decompression is a state of reduced pressure inside of a spinal disc. It is achieved through the use of a computer-aided table, specifically engineered to create negative spinal disc pressure in the patient undergoing the treatment. We've discussed the effects that gravity has on the spine over time: shrinking it and reducing the spaces between the bones. VAX-D Therapy reverses that process. Patients lay affixed to the VAX-D table while the spine is slowly pulled apart, opening up the compressed disc space and the facet joints. It increases the space within the foramen where the spinal nerves emerge and stretches the ligaments and para-spinal muscles. But the main tenant is that VAX-D Therapy has been proven to create a vacuum effect within the disc itself much like how the contraction of the diaphragm causes air to flow freely into the lungs.

Many other benefits are believed to occur along with the distraction of the joint spaces. One benefit is the rehydration of the disc with water inevitably promoting the body's natural healing processes. Another benefit is the retraction of the nucleus towards the center of the disc space. Yet another advantage is the stimulation of type IV collagen production which attaches to torn annulus fibers repairing them, making them stronger than before.

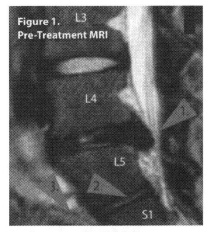
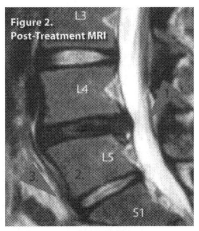

BEFORE	AFTER
1 Herniated Disc L4/L5	1 Dramatically Reduced Herniation
2 Degenerated Disc L5/S1	2 Reversal of Disc Dehydration and Increased Disc Height

VAX-D Is NOT Traction

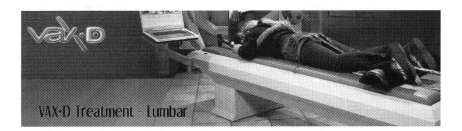

VAX·D Treatment - Lumbar

> "Traction can be expected to increase intradiscal pressure and can, therefore, aggravate a protruded, herniated or extruded disc. It is, therefore, contra-indicated for patients with herniated discs."
>
> (Source: Allan Dyer, M.D.).

The human body does not like to be pulled apart especially when the pull occurs rapidly. It responds immediately by eliciting a reflex called muscle guarding to protect itself. For this reason traction, as proven throughout its history, has shown very poor clinical outcomes with regards to the treatment of chronic LBP.

"Although pelvic traction has been used to treat patients with chronic LBP for hundreds of years, most neurosurgeons and orthopedists have not been enthusiastic about it secondary to concerns over inconsistent results and cumbersome equipment. Indeed, simple traction itself has not been highly effective; therefore, almost no pain clinics even include traction as part of their approach. A few authors, however, have reported varying techniques which widen disc spaces, decompress the discs, unload the vertebrae, reduce disc protrusion, reduce muscle spasm, separate vertebrae, and/or lengthen and stabilize the spine."

(Source: Gray FJ, Hoskins MJ. *Radiological assessment of effect of body weight traction on lumbar disc spaces.* Medical Journal of Australia 1963;2:953-954).

In the belly of your muscles you have specialized receptors known as "spindle cells" that detect changes in the length of its fibers. When you stretch a muscle spindle, a reflex elicits immediate contraction of that muscle. Think, for example, of a doctor testing your knee-jerk reaction; you cannot will yourself to prevent the inevitable kick from happening. The reflex occurs faster (1-2 milliseconds) than the blink of an eye (25 milliseconds). This acts as a protective mechanism preventing the muscle from over stretching or worse, tearing.

When the muscle guarding reflex occurs in the paraspinal muscles, it will prevent "decompression" of the spinal disc from occurring. The muscles will lock, holding the joints together. If a patient's muscles tighten during an attempted treatment, although you may feel like the treatment is working, true disc decompression will not occur. The trunk muscles are simply too strong and will hold the joints together.

VAX-D is the only device shown in clinical research to decompress the discs to negative levels.

VAX-D has patented systems in place that overcome the spindle's reflex and prevent muscle guarding from occurring during the treatment thus allowing the pressure inside the disc to decrease. The pioneers of VAX-D placed pressure-monitoring transducers into actual spinal discs of patients measuring negative intradiscal pressures down to—150mm Hg. That is significantly lower than that of resting blood pressure of 80mm Hg; resulting in re-hydration within the disc (diffusion gradient >200 mm Hg across the vertebral end plate).

VAX-D has been shown to decompress the disc space, and in clinical picture of Chronic LBP is distinguishable from conventional spinal traction. According to the literature, traction has proven to be less effective and biomechanically inadequate to produce optimal therapeutic results."

(Source: Thomas A. Gionis, MD, JD, MBA, MHA, FICS, FRCS, and Eric Groteke, DC, CCIC, *Surgical Alternatives*)

Spinal discs operate optimally within a specific range of intradiscal pressures, assuming that they are healthy. If you are young, it's typically a trauma such as a car accident or sports injury that causes a rapid increase in the intradiscal pressure that leads to a herniated disc. In the elderly, it's more often degenerative changes such as, a lifetime of pressure paired with poor lifestyle habits that causes the problems.

When treating disc bulging, herniated discs, disc protrusions, extruded discs, disc degeneration, degenerative disc disease and so on, it is important to remember: pressure is the problem! Taking that pressure off is the solution. It's a mechanical issue with a mechanical fix.

In the graph below, you will see common daily activities and the disc pressures associated with each of these activities. All activities result in a rise in intradiscal pressure(s). The more strenuous the activity, the greater the resultant pressure increase. This is exactly why Physical Therapy typically has poor clinical outcomes when treating herniated discs. In many cases, Physical Therapy can actually exacerbate patient's symptoms of chronic LBP and Sciatica.

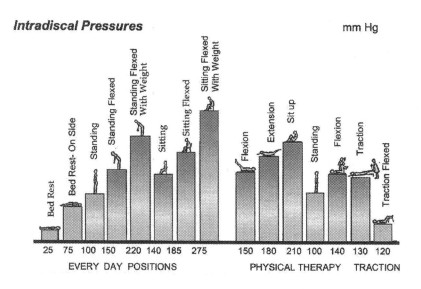

Intradiscal Pressures   mm Hg

25	75	100	150	220	140	185	275		150	180	210	100	140	130	120

EVERY DAY POSITIONS   PHYSICAL THERAPY   TRACTION

According to a study by Feline and Lund of McGill University, there is little evidence that physical therapy and physical therapy modalities provide any long-term efficacy greater than placebo.

The therapies that were examined included exercise, ultrasound, thermal agents, acupuncture, low-intensity laser therapy, electrical stimulation, and combination therapies for a variety of musculoskeletal pain conditions including chronic back pain. The authors reported, "our results suggest that none of the therapies under review cause improvements in symptoms of chronic musculoskeletal pain or in quality of life that outlast the therapy . . . including placebo."

Van den Hoogen et al published the results of a study involving 269 patients. It was concluded that receiving physical therapy was associated with a longer duration of low back pain. The authors reported, "at every moment in time, patients receiving physical therapy had a 51% less chance to recover in the following week than patients not receiving physical therapy."

Does this imply that Physical Therapy has no place at all in the treatment of chronic LBP? No. As a matter of fact, core strengthening is recommended in all of my cases. However, its implementation into a treatment plan is initiated only after the completion of the full VAX-D Treatment Protocol. While undergoing VAX-D, the goal is primarily to decrease pressure. It is counterintuitive and counterproductive to engage in activities that increase pressure during the healing process. Walking is the only activity I condone and recommend during the initial phase of my treatment plans.

"By "guts" I mean grace under pressure."

-Ernest Hemmingway {Nobel Prize winning novelist}

History Of VAX-D

Vertebral Axial Decompression (VAX-D) was founded by Dr. Alan Dyer, B.S., M.D., Ph.D. Dr. Dyer is a practitioner of Internal Medicine and is also known for his Ph.D. pioneer work on Transthoracic Cardiac Defibrillation. After retiring as a Senior Administrator and Deputy Minister of Health in Ontario, Canada in 1987, Dr. Dyer went to work expanding on early research on back pain. The late Dr. James Cyriax, an Internist and Orthopaedic Surgeon in England hypothesized that if the spine could be distracted without eliciting muscle contraction, negative pressure within the discs could be achieved thus "suctioning" any herniation(s) back into place. Dr. Dyer explored this hypothesis, but initially found that the ability to overcome muscle guarding was not an easy task.

Dr. Dyer's breakthrough was introducing a computer into the treatment that incorporates a Progressive Logarithmic Curve into the pulling force. This meant that as the tension applied increases, the speed of the tension decreases. It was so revolutionary, he was issued US patent # 6,039,737. It changed everything. Implementation of a logarithmic tension force averted the body's reflex guarding and spinal disc pressure was finally able to be decreased. What that means to a patient is symptom reduction, healing and the ability to return to a normal lifestyle.

Dr. Dyer registered his first VAX-D device with the Food & Drug Administration and was awarded three US patents and International Patents under the Patent Cooperative Treaty for the technology used in the therapy.

VAX-D: Review Of Literature

Overview:

76% of patients are pain free within just 20 treatments {1}
Patients are still pain free after four years {2}
70% success rate in patients with pain for seven years {3}

788 patients with herniated and degenerative discs;
71% were pain free {4}
Patients still pain free after six months following treatment {5 & 6}
Severe cases facing surgery achieve success {7}
Cases succeed after other methods fail {8}
VAX-D successfully decompresses nerve roots and thus leg pain {8}

Source:

1) *Efficacy of Vertabral Axial Decompression (VAX-D) on Chronic LBP: A Study of Dosage Regimen*
    Ramos G., M.D.
    Journal of Neurological Research, Volume 26, April 2004

2) *VAX-D Reduces Chronic Discogenic Chronic LBP-4 year Study*
    Odell R., MD. Ph.D, Boudreau D. DO
    Anesthesiology News, Volume 29, number 3, March 2003

3) *A Prospective Randomized Controlled Study of VAX-D and TENS for the Treatment of Chronic LBP*
    Sherry E. MD FRACS, Kitchener P., MB, BS FRANZCR, Smart R., MB, Ch.B
    Journal of Neurological Research Volume 23, Number 7, October 2001

4) *Vertebral Axial Decompression Therapy for Pain Associated with Herniated or Degenerated Discs or Facet Syndrome: An Outcome Study*
    Gose E., Ph.D, Naguszewski W., MD, Naguszewski R., MD,
    Journal of Neurological Research, Volume 20, no 3, April 1998.

5) *Short and Long Term Outcomes Following Treatment with the VAX-D Protocol for Patients with Chronic, Activity Limiting Chronic LBP*
    Beattie PF., Nelson R., Michener L., Cammaratta J., Donely J.
    Journal of Orthopedic & Sports Physical Therapy, Volume 35, Number 1, Jan 2005

6) *Outcomes after a Prone Lumbar Traction Protocol for patients with Activity-Limiting Chronic LBP: A Prospective Case series study*
    Beattie PF., Nelson R. Michener L., Cammaratta J., Donnelly J.,

Arch Phys Med Rehabil Vol89, February 2008

7) *The Fountain of Youth for the Lower Back / Acute and Chronic Case Presentations*
Varaday A. M.D., D.A.B.R., Yesak M. D.C., Elder J. B.S., M.H.A.
Dynamic Chiropractic-Vol. 26, Issue 21, October 7, 2008

8) *Dermatosomal Somatosensory Evoked Potential Demonstration Of Nerve Root Decompression After VAX-D*
Naguszewski W., MD, Naguszewski R., MD, Gose E., Ph.D
Journal of Neurological Research Volume 23, no 7, October 2001

9) *The Effects of VAX-D On Sensory Nerve Dysfunction In Patients with LBP and Radiculopathy*
Tilaro F., MD, Miskovich D. MD
Canadian Journal of Clinical Medicine Vol. 6, No 1, January 1999

10) *Effects of Vertebral Axial Decompression on Intradiscal Pressure*
Ramos G., MD, Martin W., MD,
Journal of Neurosurgery 81:350-353, 1994

11) *Prospective Randomized Study of VAX-D Therapy for Acute Low Back Distress*
Peerless S., M.D. FRCP, Meissner L., MD, FRCP
Barnett H. J.M., MD. FRCP, Stiller C.R., MD, FRCP
The John P. Robarts Institute, University Hospital at London, 1996

12) *An Industry Based, Retrospective, Cost Analysis of Vertebral Axial Decompression (VAX-D) VS. Surgery for Lumbar Disc Disease: 10 Case Studies*
David C. Duncan, MD, Don Keenan, SPHR, PhD
Sinclair Oil Corporation Study, Tulsa Oklahoma

13) *An Overview of Vertebral Axial Decompression*
Tilaro F., MD
Canadian Journal of Clinical Medicine Vol. 5, No. 1, January 1998

> "For a long time, my back pain pretty much had my life on hold. By the third session, I began to feel the pain in my feet disappear, and now I have a better outlook on life, a little more spunk in my step because I am pain free."
>
> Anastasia S.

Said simply, VAX-D Therapy works! The motto at VAX-D Medical Technologies, LLC is:

"REAL SCIENCE, REAL STUDIES, REAL RESULTS."

It is medically safe and highly effective. Below is another study on the success rate of VAX-D:

Summary Of 900 VAX-D Therapy Cases

Diagnosis	Percentage of Success
Overall Success Rate	75%
Extruded Herniated Discs	67%
Degenerative Discs	77%
Single Herniated Discs	77%
Multiple Herniated Discs	71%
Facet Syndrome	70%

VAX-D Therapy is arguably the best intervention ever developed for the treatment of chronic LBP and I encourage anyone suffering the effects of this debilitating problem to find the right doctor at the right clinic and schedule a consultation as soon as possible.

The Care

The bench mark for treatment is 20-sessions. However, the number of sessions can go up with multiple levels affected or complicating factors like IDD or Failed Back Surgery Syndrome. I've performed as many as 35 to 40-sessions on extreme but rare cases. Each session on the table can last between 30 to 40 minutes depending on your doctor's judgment.

Time on the VAX-D table is all about comfort. As you have already learned, your body does not like to be pulled. Therefore, preventing muscle guarding is crucial to a successful treatment. Each VAX-D table in my clinic is in a private room. Cell phones are asked to be onto vibrate mode while the patient is in the treatment room. The lights are switched off and soothing music is played softly in the background. The entire experience is designed to be as pleasant as possible for the patient, so much so that many patients typically fall asleep on the table during their treatment.

Many doctors use additional modalities before and after VAX-D Therapy. In my office, I utilize a wobble chair to increase circulation and warm up the tissues prior to decompression. Some clinics also use electric stimulation, infrared heat, and so on. These steps are not vital so do not think you are missing out if the doctor you visit only performs VAX-D Therapy by itself. Table time is the most important step to allow proper disc decompression to take place. If you have faith in the doctor that you visit for consultation, trust him to make the right decisions for your individual care.

My office is open Monday through Friday allowing for five consecutive days of treatment per week. Why every day? Clinical trials showed that patients who are treated 5-days per week, responded better overall compared to those who are treated less. The goal is for your body to heal while you are on the VAX-D table. The more consistently you can create that state of healing, the better the result. Playing the odds again, I recommend daily treatment for all patients. The exception can be made for those who do not have the flexibility in their schedule, but it is not recommended. Considering the facts and the proven success of VAX-D Therapy, patients are usually willing to make their VAX-D Therapy care plan their priority.

After the prescribed number of VAX-D sessions is completed, my patients are transitioned to an extended care plan for core strengthening and spinal hygiene. This phase of care is optional but highly recommended. Both core strengthening and continued disc rehydration are important post treatment. As you previously learned, becoming a PRH will pay dividends to your health in the end. RRH's who return to a predominantly sedentary and unfit lifestyle will eventually experience back pain again in the future given a long enough timeline.

Herniated and bulging spinal discs are healed by the time a patient has finished their decompression sessions. Again, VAX-D Therapy has a documented success rate of 76%. As good as that is, I have experienced even better results at my clinic. 70% of patients are still pain free after 7-years following VAX-D Therapy. That is a staggering number when compared to other mainstream interventions, which often produce a shorter duration of pain relief or no relief at all. How do the beneficial effects of VAX-D Therapy last so long? It is believed to be due to collagen production laid down onto torn disc fibers that create scar tissue. Just like the scars you may have had on your body, this tissue is stronger than the original tissue. I rarely see what proved to be a successful case needing more than the occasional "tune-up" session. The results experienced at my office last and patients are very happy long after they are discharged from my care.

Chapter 6

97% of bulging and degenerated discs are healed through Non-Surgical Spinal Decompression.

-American Academy for Pain Management {AAPM}

Spinal Decompression: The Industry

White Castle, McDonald's, Burger King and Wendy's: they all make burgers. White Castle was just the first company to make 'em. Then, followed the copy cats. Which one is the best? Who knows, who cares, right? As long as you get your fast food fix.

With the phenomenal success of VAX-D Therapy came also, the imitators. There are many companies that manufacture "decompression" tables. Unfortunately, like the knock-offs in other industries, many of the replicas are frankly not be as good as the original. Patients have come to me whose injuries were worsened following treatment in which their former doctor employed lesser quality equipment.

VAX-D is the only device that has been proven to decompress spinal discs. This is the reason why I have chosen to use them exclusively at my clinics over the years. This is not to suggest that other decompression systems fail to work. On the contrary, some of my mentors utilize other decompression systems with amazing results. I just sleep better knowing that I provide exactly the service I am claiming to provide for my patients.

With multiple providers using different decompression tables, it would appear to be difficult for a patient to choose whom to put their faith in. Much in the same fashion that you would evaluate any serious decision in life, you should choose by performing proper due diligence, listening to your intuition and by heeding the recommendations from others who found success.

Any treatment, in this case the decompression table, is secondary to the clinical judgment utilized by the physician. The decompression table alone will not ensure success. Treatment plans must be monitored with eyes wide open. I continually have to adapt to a patient's individual needs and their response to treatment. I have weekly, if not daily, interaction with my patients to gain status updates. I often extend a treatment plan by a week or more if a patient is experiencing slower progress.

Specialty Makes A Difference

My offices are Disc Specialty clinics. Each office is designed to treat herniated and degenerated disc cases with maximum efficacy. We utilize the state-of-the-art VAX-D Spinal Decompression, continued disc rehydration and core stabilization equipment, as well as ancillary products to support spinal disc patients. Offering anything less would naturally lower the outcomes for my patients and as I am sure you are aware I play the odds as much as possible.

My patients know I mean business when it comes to treating chronic LBP. My consultations are generally one full hour in duration. During this time I am also interviewing the prospective patient to gauge if they are a good fit for our office. I use my own professional judgment in evaluating what conditions will respond well to my care and which prospective patients are P.R.H.'s. That's not to say I refuse treatment to R.R.H.'s, but I do point out that they have been re-active to date and must become more pro-active if they want to achieve success in overcoming their chronic LBP. If I feel that a prospective patient does not align with our office values, I tell them candidly that I do not think that we would make a good fit for one another and refer them elsewhere.

Non-Surgical Spinal Decompression: Review Of Literature

There are studies on spinal decompression systems that do not use VAX-D equipment. However, these studies do not appear in the medical or peer reviewed literature. To date, VAX-D Medical Technologies is the only company who has demonstrated that they can produce a state of negative intradiscal pressure in patients suffering chronic LBP. However, at the end of the day, all a patient cares about is getting relief from their unrelenting pain. Although I exclusively use VAX-D at my clinic, the table is only part of the equation in a successful treatment regimen and not to sound redundant, I do know clinics using other systems with comparable results. I would be remiss if I did not share the success rates reported with other equipment.

"Results showed 86% of the 219 patients who completed the therapy reported immediate resolution of symptoms, while 84% remained pain-free 90-days post treatment. Physical examination findings showed improvement in 92% of the 219 patients, and the remained intact in 89% of these cases 90 days after treatment."

The cost for successful non-surgical therapy is less than a tenth of the cost of surgery.

"Alteration of normal kinetics is the most prevalent cause of chronic LBP and disc disruption and thus it is vital to maintain homeostasis in and around the spinal disc."

{Source: Thomas A. Gionis, MD, JD, MBA, MHA, FICS, FRCS, and Eric Groteke, DC, CCIC, *Surgical Alternatives*}

"Eighty-six percent of ruptured intervertebral disc (RID) patients achieved "good" (50—89% improvement) to "Excellent" (90-100%

improvement) results with decompression. Sciatica and back pain were relieved. Of the facet arthrosis patients, 75% obtained "good" to "Excellent" results with decompression."

{Source: C. Norman Shealy, MD, PhD, and Vera Borgmeyer, RN, MA. *Decompression, Reduction and Stabilization of the Lumbar Spine: A Cost-Effective Treatment for Lumbosacral Pain.* American Journal of Pain Management Vol. 7 No. 2 April 1997}

"Serial MRI of 20 patients treated with the decompression table shows in our study up to 90% reduction of subligamentous nucleus herniation in 10 of 14. Some rehydration occurs detected by T2 and proton density signal increase. Torn annulus repair seen in all."

{Source: Eyerman, Edward M.D. *Simple pelvic traction gives inconsistent relief to herniated lumbar disc suffers.* Journal of Neuroimaging. Paper presented to the American Society of Neuroimaging. Orlando, Florida 2-26-98}

When your body triggers the warning light that your spine is degenerating, Non-Surgical Spinal Decompression statistically offers you the best chances of reversing the process.

86% of patients with herniated or ruptured discs are healed through Non-Surgical Spinal Decompression.

-American Journal of Pain Management {AJPM}

So Why Haven't I Heard Of VAX-D Or Spinal Decompression Before?

There's an old saying that goes, "If all you got in your toolbox is a hammer, every problem looks like a nail." This adage is especially true when it comes to visiting a doctor's office.

Upon reciting their Hippocratic oath, every doctor has a genuine desire to care, to help and above all, to do no harm. You may hear stories about a few bad apples from time to time as in any industry or profession, but it is my belief that the majority of doctors are true altruists. To that end, doctors usually will not let you leave their office without offering you some form of help any way they can. Patients feel unsatisfied, even jilted when they give up their time and spend their money to schedule a doctor's visit and leave with nothing. Therefore, doctors simply offer their best option, one readily available in their personal toolbox.

VAX-D is a business within itself. The equipment is very expensive. The staffing and other overhead is exorbitant. This makes entering into a VAX-D "business" more cost-prohibitive. The economics can be too challenging for busy physicians to involve themselves with VAX-D. There are less road blocks to offering other treatment options that comes with lower expenses, lower management challenges, while at the same time offering significantly higher revenue.

Another reason you may not have heard of VAX-D is that studies have shown that treatments are directly proportionate to the number of physicians offering said treatments. The occurrence rate for lower back surgery correlates to the number of surgeons who perform that surgery. It has nothing to do at all with the success of that procedure but more so on the numbers of physicians who are certified to perform such surgeries.

Don't get discouraged and give up hope. There are many specialty non-surgical spinal decompression clinics in the US and throughout other countries in the world. You will find one that fits your needs with doctors dedicated to offering the best spinal care or disc care, today.

How Much Is This Going To Cost Me?

A typical care plan for the treatment of chronic LBP that incorporates the use of non-surgical spinal decompression can range anywhere from $2,000 to $10,000. In rare cases, the cost could be higher. Treatment sessions often include additional modalities such as heat, electric stimulation, spinal adjustments, proprioceptive wobble chairs or soft tissue massage. In addition, after the decompression sessions are completed, recommendations are usually made for patients to strengthen their core muscles and continually rehydrate the spinal discs for up to 5 months, once or twice per week. Insurance coverage for spinal decompression varies from state to state. In Pennsylvania, where my clinic operates, VAX-D Therapy is covered when you are injured in a motor vehicle accident only. For the most part however, the spinal decompression component to a care plan is an elective procedure and thus, paid for by the patient. Major medical insurances often cover most of the additional expenses associated with a full treatment regimen.

Out-of-pocket expenses are usually less than or equal to out-of-pocket costs, such as the co-pay/co-insurance to have surgery. The least expensive care plan written at my office costs $4,000 for 20-visits of VAX-D Therapy and is paid for by the patient. We provide patient financing through an affiliate bank as a courtesy to our patients as do most other non-surgical spinal decompression clinics. Some clinics even offer interest free loans.

I perform hundreds of consultations every year. Every patient without fail asks, "If VAX-D Therapy works so well, why won't my insurance cover it?"

The short answer is: they don't have to! That's right, most insurance companies consider VAX-D Therapy an elective procedure. More and more procedures today are facing the same issues. Lasik eye surgery, gastric bypass, and most cosmetic procedures fall under the same insurance guidelines even though you may need to have these procedures performed to maintain your health.

I personally know many talented doctors leaving their profession to open pizza restaurants due to the over regulation and under reimbursement in today's health care system. It is a terrible feeling for me to see my colleagues leave their profession because of all the red tape insurance companies throw their way. Here's what I can tell you for sure. If you are expecting a corporation to do what is in your best interest as opposed to their own, chances are you'll die waiting.

Chapter 7

"If all medicines in the world were thrown into the sea, it would be all the better for mankind and all the worse for the fishes."

-Oliver Wendell Holmes, Sr. {American physician & poet}

The Choice Is Yours

Medication

I believe it would be difficult to find anyone, in today's society, other than the Big Pharmaceutical companies themselves, to disagree with the following statement: "The United States is overly medicated!" Let me state clearly that I am not categorically anti-medicine nor I am anti-surgery. In the event that I should ever be admitted into an emergency room following some horrific accident, I want the best medicine and the most advanced surgery at my disposal.

Medications are believed to have been around since the dawn of mankind with pre-historic man using plants to treat illness. The majority of medications were found to be largely ineffective up to the 20th century. However, following a substantial investment in creating medicine, there have been tremendous gains in knowledge in the fields of chemistry, bio-chemistry and physiology that makes drugs a main staple in any physician's toolbox today.

Despite showing that medications do produce a desired effect on the body's chemistry, there is a lack of evidence supporting that medications make us healthier as a whole. There is evidence supporting their use for acute LBP but supporting data for their use in the treatment of chronic LBP is limited, at best. With this fact widely accepted, why is it that medications continue to be prescribed in copious amounts after three months? It is because it is the easiest tool to take out of the toolbox, it costs the least and there may not be a substitute your physician has readily available.

I believe oral medications are unlikely to resolve your chronic LBP long term. Oral medications merely mask the pain as medications are often designed to do.

There are 106,000 deaths annually due to prescription drugs even when they are prescribed correctly.

-Journal of the American Medical Association {JAMA}

All drugs can have adverse side effects accompanying the intended effect. As much as we would like to believe that modern medicine is a perfected art form in the treatment of a disease, the statistic proves it is not.

Adverse reactions to "Properly Prescribed" drugs are the 4th leading cause of death in the United States. Only heart disease, cancer and stroke will kill more Americans than drugs prescribed by medical doctors.

-Newsweek

Offering little more than a temporary solution for the treatment of chronic LBP, you may want to revisit the topic of prescription medications and their prolonged usage with your doctor if your LBP persists past 90-days.

E.S.I. And Other Spinal Injections

There are multiple spinal injections your doctor may order to help you cope with chronic LBP. One of the more common is Epidural Steroid Injection (ESI). ESI's are often prescribed if oral medication and physical therapy has been unsuccessful in treating the symptoms of chronic LBP. Most of my consult patients have already had at least a series of three ESI's prior to seeking my help. ESI treatments often reduce inflammation temporarily. Virtually all studies have shown a lack of their efficacy after one year.

The British Journal of Medicine reported that epidural injections of cortisone are largely ineffective at relieving chronic and severe low back pain.

Like oral medications, injections can have adverse side effects from bleeding and infections to neurological damage and meningitis.

Local anesthetics are often injected into the soft tissues, more specifically the trigger points. One double-blind study compared local anesthetic injections to saline and reported no long-term benefit.

Corticosteroids are sometimes injected into the muscles and facet joints. Facet injections were shown to have no beneficial difference when compared to saline injections after one month in a controlled trial.

Does this imply that injections have no place in the treatment of chronic LBP? No. Doctors on my team sometimes utilize injections (facet injections mostly) when a patient's inflammation is so great it causes antalgia. We also use injections when algometry or pain mapping shows a very low tolerance to pressure. If pain limits a patient's ability to lay prone or supine comfortably, injections are ordered to reduce the inflammation. But, this is done only to relieve their discomfort long enough for them to receive VAX-D Therapy without issue. Typically, the pain experienced by these patients is manageable after two to three days. They do not need to be injected from that point onward.

Spine Surgery

It is absolutely amazing what surgeons can do today. A skilled surgeon can literally put the pieces back together saving a life. There is no doubt that the United States has the best emergency care systems in the world. But, we are talking about emergency care, not surgery prescribed for the treatment of chronic LBP. Unfortunately, the statistics for lumbar spine surgeries are bleak.

> "Each day I wake up without having to deal with the excruciating pain I once had is a day worth living. I am thankful that I got the help I needed without the extremes of surgery.
>
> Jerry B.

51% of back surgeries are unnecessary.

-New England Journal of Medicine

53% of all lumbar surgeries fail to produce relief of symptoms.

-International Orthopedics

Lately, I've come across patients who romanticize having surgery for their chronic LBP. They are usually RRH's who like to believe that only a miraculous surgical intervention performed by only the best doctor can save them. It could be shear hopelessness that brought them to this place or some underlying psychological issue.

As talented as surgeons can be at their best, we should not readily turn to surgery lightly. For all of the advancements in equipments, techniques and knowledge, there will always be risks in any kind of surgery. Spinal fusion surgery incurs a hospital bill in excess of $34,000 that does not even include the doctor's fees. This kind of surgery comes at an exorbitant price tag and affords you little odds of success.

Faith's Story

"I was involved in an auto accident this past December and injured my back. An MRI showed that I had a herniated disc among other problems. After months of pain, my lower back pain worsened to an unbelievable degree. The pain was absolutely terrible, so bad that I could not often get out of bed. Just when I thought that the back pain could not get worse, walking up the stairs one day I felt this horrible shooting pain go down my left leg and into my foot. My left foot was totally numb.

At this time, the Neurosurgeon said that my only option would be surgery.

My disc ruptured and therefore it was important that we do something as soon as possible to avoid further complications. I was miserable, could barely get out of bed, walk, sit comfortably, work, drive, pretty much . . . I could barely live. I hated how I felt, but more than that I hated the idea of surgery.

A while back, my fiancée and I had seen a channel 3 news documentary and learned about the Non-Surgical Spinal Decompression system. The rest is history! The first week, I felt better. I started to have less pain in my leg, some feeling came back to my foot, and the back pain almost completely subsided. The second week, even after me overdoing it that weekend, I felt a little bit better again. After my fourth week, I was pain free. I am living a normal life again . . ."

Faith A.

Hubert L. Rosomoff, M.D., Medical Director of the Comprehensive Pain and Rehabilitation Center at the University of Miami School of Medicine, called for a moratorium on back surgeries in February 2001. Dr. Rosomoff stated that, a doctor "can eliminate 99 percent of surgical cases." He further estimates the incidence of surgery at only one of 500.

There are states, such as Illinois that make lumbar spine surgery illegal in the absence of cauda equine syndrome. CES is characterized by incontinence following loss of function of the lumbar plexus. I refer any CES cases for surgery.

The US performs 40% more back surgeries than any other countries. As noted earlier, the increase in procedures is commensurate to the number of surgeons in that country; it is not a relationship based on a stellar rate of success.

A German neurologist named Henrik Weber conducted a study on patients experiencing sciatica associated with disc herniations. These patients were assigned to an operative group and a non-operative group. After 4-10 years there was no recorded difference in improvement.

Surgery as a successful treatment for chronic LBP quite simply does not have a good track record.

> "We all have a bias for action. Both doctors and patients hate the idea of just wait and see, or try something that doesn't seem very dramatic."
>
> {Source: Dr. Rick Deyo JAMA Feb 13}

Failed Back Syndrome (failed surgery) can occur in as many as 10%-40% of patients who received some type of lumbar spine surgery.

—American Academy of Pain Medicine {AAPM}

President Barak Obama warns us that, "We are paying more, getting less, and going broke." President Obama also stated that health care reform legislation is needed to prevent the United States from further financial decay. President Obama went further to declare that, "Today, we are spending over $2 trillion per year on health care; almost 50% more per person than the next most costly nation."

"Harvard University found that 62% of all personal bankruptcies filed in 2007 was the result of unpaid medical bills. 78% of those who filed for bankruptcies had health insurance!

Not surprisingly, some of the most numerous medical malpractice lawsuits in the United States are those relating to spinal surgery!

Malpractice is the 3rd leading cause of preventable death.

1) **Cigarette**
2) **Alcohol**
3) **Medical Malpractice**
4) **Traffic Fatalities**
5) **Hand Guns**

$\qquad\qquad\qquad\qquad\qquad\qquad$ **-Harvard University Study**

It's been reported that over 3,000 Americans die every single week due to surgery gone awry. America also performs more surgeries than any other country with a total of over 60 million surgeries in 2006. That's about one in every five citizens.

Most chronic LBP patients can be considered "good candidates" for having spine surgery. Surgeries of all kinds are performed every day but there will always be inherent risks and permanent changes no matter how minor the surgeries performed may be. You cannot undo surgery!

I do not enjoy having to refer any patient for surgery. With that being said, no matter what my personal position is, I cannot get around the fact there are cases such as CES that warrant the risks of surgery. I refer all such emergency cases without hesitation. But that number is a miniscule percentage. These emergency cases usually involve patients who are hospitalized and rarely visit an independent practitioner's office.

Spine Surgery Is Not The Only Option

If you've been told that you need surgery and that it's the only thing that will help you, I urge you to consider every possible alternative first, then again a second time, and one final time for good measure. The surgeons will still be there, knife in hand, if you are truly left with no option or you if progress to emergency status.

> "I can't believe the quality in my life since the treatments. I can walk 1 or 2 miles a time, stand for periods of time without pain and no longer need a gel cushion at work to sit on. I am recommending this to everyone! My x-rays definitely show this works.
>
> Hugh G.

Chapter 8

Additional Recommendations

Spinal Lift

During the Disc Rehabilitation portion of our care plan (the 20 or more daily VAX-D Therapy visits), I prescribe ancillary products to help maximize the overall effects of the treatment. These products are part of our system of spinal health care and therefore, mandatory for acceptance into our program. These products are proven to be highly effective features to our care. They are irreplaceable assets to the process of healing degenerated, compressed spines. One of the products I utilize is the Spinal Lift.

The Spinal Lift is an ambulatory spinal air traction belt made for our system of spinal decompression. It is a soft girdle like belt that is worn snuggly on the waist. Wearing a crude support belt alone does very little to treat chronic LBP and in the case of a herniated disc, the belt can exacerbate the condition. The Spinal Lift is a patented, Medicare approved device that pumps 15 pounds of air into the internal vertical air expansion cells helping to lift the spine 3.5 inches thus reducing the spinal pressure. I fit the belt onto the patient immediately following their VAX-D Therapy session. Then, they must wear it for 2 ½ hours. This extends a patient's daily treatment time from 30-45 minutes to nearly three hours. This provides 60 hours per month of reduced pressure unloading the spine! You can calculate the cumulative effect this has over the course of the treatment.

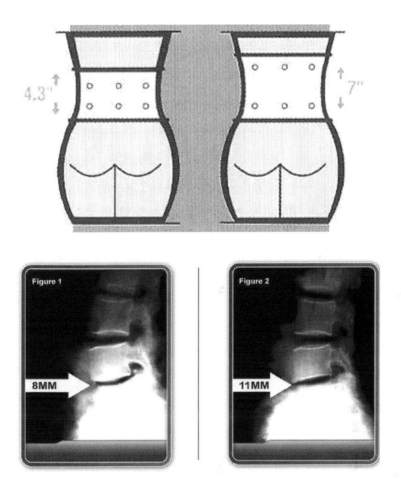

As you can see in the above x-ray, an increase of up to 2mm of height can be achieved between the vertebrae and that's only in one spinal level! The spine has five lumbar vertebrae. For the patient wearing the spinal lift, this simply means one thing: pain relief. They report feeling stronger when they wear the spinal lift and more stabilized when walking and performing chores.

Spinal Lift also comes with detachable, rigid anterior and posterior panels that offer extra spinal stabilization for patients experiencing a high level of pain. As a patient's treatment progresses and their pain decreases, the rigid panels can be easily removed for a more comfortable soft lumbar sacral orthosis that allows for greater flexibility.

Features of the Spinal Lift

- Patented vertical expansion air cells
- 1600 Gauss medical grade magnets
- Helps maintain proper lumbar posture, supporting the natural curve of the lumbar spine
- Waterproof and machine washable

Patients rarely complain and they feel great wearing it. I have sold numerous Spinal Lift belts to patients who were physically unable to make a visit to my office and they have reported tremendous pain relief.

"I have been using Spinal Lift for about 18 months now. I first injured my back over 17 years ago when I fell on a ceramic tile floor. The fall caused my L5 disc to bulge. Since then my lower back had gotten worse as my discs had degenerated. No doctor or surgeon could help me. Weekly visits to my chiropractor were all that was saving me. During this time I never stopped looking for a remedy. Every three months or so I would use Google to search for various key words for back pain remedies. Then finally I found Spinal Lift and I have been wearing it religiously since. I love it! It works! I can definitely tell my back is finally healing. I am no longer in pain and am even able to start exercising again. I estimate that in another 6 months my back will be totally healed.

Kathy B.

Indication for the use of the Spinal Lift

- Bulging/Herniated Disc
- Disc Protrusion
- Extruded Disc
- Disc Degeneration
- Degenerative Disc Disease
- Loss of Disc Signal
- Disc Desiccation

- IDD
- Facet Arthrosis
- Spondylolisthesis
- Foraminal Stenosis
- Sciatica
- Spinal Stenosis (secondary to disc herniation)
- Nerve Root Compression
- Great for strenuous jobs requiring heavy lifting and/or long hours driving.
- Relaxes muscle spasms and muscle cramps.

Spinal Lift Cervical Model

Just as VAX-D Therapy can be performed on the same conditions that exist in the neck, there is also a cervical Spinal Lift model. It's easy to use and can offer you relief from:

- Chronic Migraines
- Chronic Neck Pain
- Bulging/Herniated Disc
- Disc Protrusion
- Extruded Disc
- Disc Degeneration
- Degenerative Disc Disease
- Loss of Disc Signal
- Disc Desiccation
- IDD
- Facet Arthrosis
- Foraminal Stenosis
- Spinal Stenosis (secondary to disc herniation)
- Nerve Root Compression

Core Strengthening & Disc Re-Hydration

When patients are discharged from their active VAX-D Therapy plan they often ask "Now that I am feeling better, what can I do to prevent myself from ever feeling the pain again?"

Widely considered the expert on the Science of Human Wellness, Dr. James L. Chestnut's book, *Innate Physical Fitness & Spinal Hygiene*, introduces us to the concept of Movement Deficiency Syndrome. Dr. Chestnut proves through evidence-based science that, "Exercise is a required nutrient for homeostasis and our genes are programmed to need it in order to create healthy cell function throughout our ecosystem of cells."

We as a society are less physically fit than our hunter-gatherer ancestors. A weaker body compounded with chronic LBP usually limits physical activity even further thus producing a De-Conditioning Syndrome.

I always recommend strengthening the core muscles to stabilize a weak spine after the healing process has taken place following VAX-D Therapy. In addition to strengthening the spine, I further recommend continually rehydrating the spinal discs. These procedures are performed by the patient on specialty equipment in my office once or twice a week, for three to five additional months post VAX-D Therapy.

Some patients initially feel that they can do this on their own at home, but I advise them to begin exercise in my office for at least two months. Strengthening the deep muscles of the spine, specifically those surrounding the spinal discs, is more difficult than training the superficial muscle groups at your local gym. As such, it is best performed on specialty equipment and under a doctor's supervision. If they are feeling confident after the two month mark, I will allow them to perform it on their own. I provide specific exercise under these conditions and can arrange for the purchase of inexpensive specialty equipment constructed for home usage.

The goal here is to strengthen the core while gaining full range of motion in the spine allowing for the patient to return to an active lifestyle. I expect a pain free outcome for every case I accept. VAX-D Therapy followed by a supportive post treatment plan does offer a much better chance of success than other treatment options, statistically speaking.

Nothing is more fulfilling in my work than the gratitude I receive from my patients. Listening to successful patients share in their own words how VAX-D Therapy literally changed their lives makes me fully aware that I have accomplished my goals. I am truly blessed that they allow me to help them.

To hear some of these amazing stories first hand visit **www. ibecameabeliever.com**. These are not my personal cases but they are actual Spinal Decompression patients, not actors.

Posture 101

Poor posture is one of the greatest stressors on the spine that adds to its premature degeneration. We are not designed from a bioengineering perspective to sit or stand for 8-hours per day with limited movement, especially in poor positions. We are designed to hunt and gather; we are made to be in motion. Slouching postures with rounded backs and dropped heads exponentially increases strain on the spine.

Donald D Harrison, M.S., D.C. wrote the book on spinal biomechanics called *The Ideal Normal Upright Static Human Spine*. Mathematical models show the design that channels the weight of your body parts against gravitational force throughout the entire body with maximum efficiency.

"Equilibrium equations dictate the center of mass of the skull, thorax, pelvis, vertebrae, knees, and ankles must lie in the median-sagittal plane."

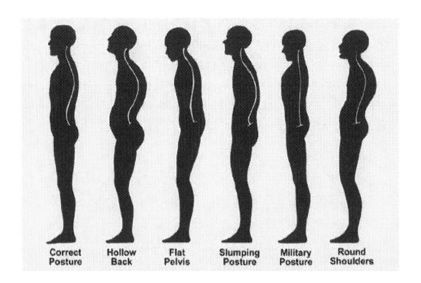

| Correct Posture | Hollow Back | Flat Pelvis | Slumping Posture | Military Posture | Round Shoulders |

Optimal posture with optimal spinal curves as seen in the illustration has proven to be very efficient. It's similar to the mathematics used in constructing a building. Centers of gravity over centers of gravity with shock absorbers (the spinal curves) strategically placed. Poor construction leads to eventual structural failure or in the body, decay.

I educate all of my patients on proper posture once their spinal discs are healed and they progress into the core-strengthening program. It is a crucial piece in maintaining a healthy spine long term. Even those who are not suffering from herniated and premature disc degeneration can benefit greatly from restoring optimal posture. Optimal function always follows optimal structure. I recommend that you seek evaluation with a certified CBP practitioner at **www.cbppatient.com**. These doctors can restore your spine to a normal biomechanical alignment.

> "I would recommend this machine to anyone who has had any type of back problems for a period of time. My only regret through this process is "I wish I knew about this machine two years ago!"
>
> Katrina F.

Ergonomics is defined as the applied science of equipment design, as for the workplace, intended to maximize productivity by reducing operator fatigue and discomfort. There is a wonderful book I use as a resource when educating patients on sitting, standing and lying techniques. *8 Steps to a Pain-Free Back*, by Ester Gokhale, L.Ac. Gokhale beautifully uses photos and illustrations to easily teach anyone proper form. Add this one to your library list and you'll feel less stress as a result. **www.egwellness.com**.

Chapter 10

Conclusion

Say YES And DECOMPRESS

As they say, Knowledge is Power. It can be confusing for one to figure out what treatment is best suited for one's self. You may come across information and literature that can be poorly presented or outright erroneous.

I have been successfully treating chronic LBP for over a decade. For many of the people who seek my consultation, I am their last hope. They have tried medication, injections and many have had surgery and yet they still suffer from pain. There is little I have to do to convince them to try VAX-D Therapy because they are still in pain and want, or more appropriately, need a solution. They can judge for themselves that I am deeply committed to their healing. They can witness the evidence of success in treating chronic LBP cases all around my office. Active patients are eager to share their experiences when they have found a successful treatment, particularly when past treatments had failed them, both physically and emotionally.

My goal in writing *DECOMPRESS: Live Your Life Free From Back Pain* is to share with you the facts and let you judge for yourself if this type of treatment is the right option for you. My office is about educating the public above all else. I don't "sell" care to patients. I present facts along with some of my personal opinions and leave them to make the most educated decision they can make for themselves. Should it turn out that VAX-D Therapy is not a fit for you and/or your lifestyle, I still want you to have the best information available. I promise you at the very least that you'll have better peace of mind with any decision you choose if you know all the options. I only want what is best for you and you are the only one who can make that choice for yourself.

As Jack Canfield puts it, you are 100% responsible for your life's choices. You are the one who must take action. You have to become more Pro-Active Regarding your Health. Being re-active in nature does not lead to better health. If you have read this far, you've already taken the first step toward a solution for your chronic LBP by educating yourself. The physical work should now follow. First by healing, than by strengthen your body.

You have little to lose and everything to gain in scheduling a consultation with a certified VAX-D provider. You can always return to pain medications if that is the way you chose to live. I only want you to know that options exist and in my opinion and experience, there is a much better option in the care plan I recommended for you throughout this book.

Regardless of what choices you make, I hope that you find a solution for your pain. Because living in pain is not living at all.

References

Acute low back problems in adults: assessment and treatment. US Department of Health and Human Services; 1994 Dec; Rockville, MD.

American Chronic Pain Association, "Facts about Chronic Pain,"

American Chronic Pain Association, "Facts About Chronic Pain," Louis Harris and associates survey for business and Health Magazine, June 1996.

Anderson GB. Epidemiological features of chronic low-back pain. Lancet. 1999; 354: 581-585.

Back Pain Patient Outcomes Assessment Team (BOAT). In MEDTEP Update, Vol. 1 Issue 1, Agency for Health Care Policy and Research, Rockville, MD, Summer 1994.

Bigos S., Bower O. Braen G, et al. Acute Low Back Problems in Adults. Rockville, MD: Agency for Health Care Policy and Research, Public Health Service, US Dept of Health and Human Services; 1994. Clinical Practice Guideline 14, AHCPR Publication 95-0642.

Binod Prasad Shah, M.D., *Current Therapeutic Options for Chronic Low Back Pain: A Focus on Nonsurgical Approaches.*

Cunningham LS, Kelsey JL. Epidemiology of musculoskeletal impairments and associated disability, Am J Public Health 1984;74:574-579.

David W. Chow, M.D., *Non-Surgical Spine Care and Pain Management.*

Dr. Doug Burton, Surgeon and Senior Spine Research Professor at the University of Kansas Medical Center.

Gary Arthritis Foundation Claxton, Vice President of the Henry J. Kaiser Family Foundation, which monitors health care spending.

Gray FJ, Hoskins MJ. Radiological assessment of effect of body weight traction on lumbar disc spaces. Medical Journal of Australia 1963;2:953-954.

Interview with Allen Dyer, *Where It All Began*, The American Chiropractor, March 2008.

Karen Springen, Price of Pain, Newsweek.

Liebenson CS. Pathogenesis of chronic back pain. J Manipulative Physical Therapy 1992; 15:299-308.

Loeser, J (1996) Editorial comment: *Back pain in the work place II*

Long DM, Ben Debba M. Torgerson WS. Et al. Persistent back pain and sciatica in the United States: Patient Characteristics. J Spinal Discors 1996. 9:40-58.

Mayo Clinic http://www.mayoclinic.com/health/back_pain/DS00171

McCraig LF. National Hospital Ambulatory Medical Care Survey: 1992 emergency department summary. Advance data from vital and health statistics; no.245. Hyattsville, MD: National Center for Health Statistics, 1994.

Murphy PL, Volinn E. is occupational Chronic LBP on the rise? Spine.1994; 24:691-697.

National Center for Health Statistics. Health, United States 2005, with chart book on trends in the health of Americans. www.cdc.gov/nchs/data/hus/hus07.pdf#contents. Accessed February 26, 2008.

National Data—Yeume Luo, Duke.

New England Journal of Medicine, 1988.

Nicolas E. Walsh, *Back Pain Matters*, Karger Gazette issue no.65.

NIOSH Technical Report

Norman Shealy, MD, PhD, and Pierre L. LeRoy, M.D. *New Concept in Back Pain Management: Decompression, Reduction and Stabilization.*

Richard A. Deyo., M.D., M.P.H., and James N. Weinstein, D.O. Chronic LBP. New England Journal of Medicine February; 2001.

Richard A. Deyo., M.D., M.P.H., Back Pain Patient Outcome Assessment Team (BOAT), Agency for Health Care Research and Quality. Summer,1994.

Richard Staehler, M.D., *Epidural Steroid Injection Pain Relief Success Rates.*

Sheldon EA, Bird SR, Smugar SS, Tershakovec AM. Correlation of measures of pain, function and overall response. Spine. 2008;33:533-538.

Snook, Stover. The costs of back pain in industry, occupational back pain, State-of-art review. Spine 1987; 2(No.1):1-4.

Stan Mendenhall, editor and publisher of Orthopedic Network News.

Stan Mendenhall, Orthopedic Network News

Thomas A. Gionis and Eric Groteke, *Spinal Decompression*

Vallfors B. Acute, Subacute and Chronic LBP: Clinical Symptoms, Absenteeism and Working Environment. Scan J. Rehab Med Supply 1985; 11: 1-98.

WebMD.com, *Pathophysiology of Chronic Back Pain*

www2.arthritis.org/conditions/DiseaseCenter/back_pain.asp

www.allaboutbackpain.com/html/spine_general/spine_general_injections.html

www.bigbackpain.com/epiduralsteroidinjection.html

www.evolutionhealth.com/Inversion_Therapy/Gravity_Inversion.html

www.medicalmalpractice.com/resources/medical-malpractice/medical-malpractice-injuries/laminectomy-error-lawsuit.html

www.orthopedics.about.com/cs/backpain/a/epiduralsteroid.html

Secret To A Life Time Of Better Health

<u>Step 1</u>

Eat the foods nature intended you to eat.

Step 2

Work your body every day.

Step 3

Maintain a healthy mental attitude.

Perform these simple recommendations at the same time, for a period of time. Your body will then express health, as designed.

"Every human being is the author of their own health or disease"
-Buddha {Enlightened Spiritual Teacher}